Dash Diet

I0082511

The Ultimate Beginner's Guide To Dash Diet to Naturally Lower Blood Pressure & Proven Weight Loss Recipes

By *Louise Jiannes*

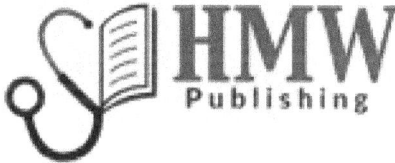

For more great books visit:

HMWPublishing.com

Get another book for Free

I want to thank you for purchasing this book and offer you another book (just as long and valuable as this book), "Health & Fitness Mistakes You Don't Know You're Making", completely free.

Visit the link below to signup and receive it:

www.hmwpublishing.com/gift

In this book, I will break down the most common health & fitness mistakes, you are probably committing right now, and I will reveal how you can easily get in the best shape of your life!

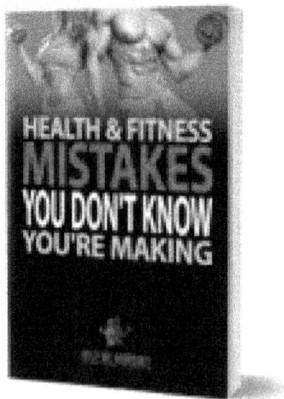

In addition to this valuable gift, you will also have an opportunity to get our new books for free, enter giveaways, and receive other valuable emails from me. Again, visit the link to sign up:

www.hmwpublishing.com/gift

Table of Contents

INTRODUCTION

In today's modern, all of us are concerned about our health more than ever before. This is due to the increase in diseases, viruses and other things that can affect how we live and how well we can continue to live the way that we want or need to. As a result of this, many new great diets have come to be. One of the most popular, if not the most popular is the DASH Diet. The DASH Diet is aimed for the prevention and cure of common diseases such as hypertension and diabetes by especially lowering sodium intake, sugars, and fats. Although it is designed for this, it has proved to be very effective for weight loss, help lower risk of osteoporosis, kidney problems, and even cancer.

Also, before you get started, I recommend you **joining our email newsletter** to receive updates on any upcoming new book releases or promotions. You can sign-up for free, and as a bonus, you will receive a free gift. Our "*Health & Fitness Mistakes*

You Don't Know You're Making" book! This book has been written to demystify, expose the top do's and don'ts and to finally equip you with the information you need to get in the best shape of your life. Due to the overwhelming amount of mis-information and lies told by magazines and self-proclaimed "gurus", it's becoming harder and harder to get reliable information to get in shape. As opposed to having to go through dozens of biased, unreliable and un-trustworthy sources to get your health & fitness information. Everything you need to help you has been broken down in this book for you to easily follow and to immediately get results to achieve your desired fitness goals in the shortest amount of time.

Once again, to join our free email newsletter and to receive a free copy of this valuable book, please visit the link and signup now:

www.hmwpublishing.com/gift

CHAPTER 1: THE MOST EFFECTIVE DIET THAT YOU SHOULD KNOW

Nowadays, tips about losing weight are everywhere. Especially on social media, there are so many short videos and photos that advise on the specifics of dieting. However, these health suggestions are unreliable. Despite their invalidity, a lot of people still take them as truth. It is a waste of time, if not dangerous, for individuals who quickly adapt to what the internet tells them. You will be spared from this nonsense however because you will be learning about the real deal in dieting. It is the single most effective diet that you should straight go to instead of doing trial and errors with other trending methods. We only have one body and one life. We cannot afford to experiment with our health.

What is the DASH Diet?

DASH diet is not just another baseless social trend. It is well researched and studied. In fact, it is endorsed by doctors and other organizations such as The National Heart, Lung, and Blood Institute, the America Heart Association, the Dietary Guidelines for Americans, and the US guidelines for treatment of high blood pressure. DASH diet is a dietary approach that helps prevent hypertension, lessen cholesterol amount in one's body, improve insulin production, and even lowers blood pressure. DASH diet goes beyond the laymen's advice of decrease sodium content in one's diet. It goes as far as designing its eating program of low fat or nonfat dairy, more fruits, and more vegetables to lower blood pressure. It stresses the importance of eating less refined grains and eat more of whole grains. DASH diet is rich in fiber, potassium, magnesium, and calcium.

Originally, DASH diet is designed to lower blood pressure and not a weight loss eating program.

Mainly, it contains whole grains, fish, poultry, nuts, beans, lean meats, and moderate fat. DASH diet is comparable to the Mediterranean diet because it has particular guidelines. Due to the low sodium content of this diet on par with loads of vitamins and minerals, it does not only lower blood pressure, but it helps reduce cholesterol as well.The DASH Diet is simple and emphasizes on.

• Eating more fruits, veggies, and low-fat dairy foods

• Lessen the intake of foods that are high in cholesterol, trans-fats and saturated fat.

• Eat a moderate amount of whole grains, poultry, fish, and nuts.

• Limit intake of sweets, sodium, sugary drinks and red meats.

Why was the DASH Diet created?

The DASH Diet was not originally made to reduce

unwanted fats in your body. It was however created to help people such as ourselves to live healthier and support us have lower chances of getting diseases. To be specific, this kind of diet can help you prevent hypertension, reduce cholesterol, improve insulin sensitivity and it has been proven to lower blood pressure to a healthy level. Also, this diet became more popular due to the added benefit of actually losing weight while still eating a decent amount of food that is chosen more carefully. As mentioned earlier, you can even eat meat to maintain a balanced protein intake. This will help you keep or gain muscle while losing weight in the process. Another thing that this diet does is it enables you to avoid eating "empty carbs."

Empty carbs are carbohydrates that lack the right amount of fiber. Refined grain carbohydrates are considered to be unhealthy in that sense. Some of these are food made from white flour such as cakes, cookies, white bread, etc. Bad carbohydrates can also come from taking in soft drinks, alcohol and even white rice. It is better to eat whole grains, nuts, vegetables, fruits and other things that are sources of good carbohydrates. It is important to mention that this diet is not a "low-carb" diet, it just makes you eat the good kinds of carbohydrates because carbohydrates are the body's primary source of energy thus making it very important for proper functioning.

How does DASH Diet work?

In the years 2011 up to 2015, DASH Diet has been ranked by the US News and World Report as the number one diet. Many people followed this diet. Natural remedies and a healthy diet are believed to be the best prevention and cure for illnesses including hypertension and diabetes. The effect of DASH Diet to one's body is similar to what pricey prescriptions do. Medicines can lower blood pressure and lessen the likelihood of someone experiencing a heart attack, stroke, or heart failure. The DASH diet has a similar effect on your health.

Even though you do not have hypertension and other illnesses, it is still advisable to follow the DASH Diet to prevent yourself from acquiring diseases. If you suspect yourself to be suffering from hypertension, consult your doctor immediately and inquire if you can just follow the DASH Diet instead of taking medications. On the other hand, if you are someone with hypertension and is already on prescriptions, talk to your doctor whether you can switch to DASH Diet and gradually take yourself off the medication.

Who should be on the DASH diet?

The DASH Diet also adapts to the person's personal preferences in the sense that it also has a diet plan for people who are vegetarians, omnivores or people who want an all natural [meaning additive free] diet. There is even an option to create your DASH Diet weight loss plan with the help of their books "The DASH Diet Action Plan" and "The DASH Diet Weight Loss Solution" Basically; anyone and everyone can use it. Young or old, broad or slim. However, you may be there is no doubt that you can, and you should follow this diet plan if you want to achieve positive results. Additionally, it is recommended for people who are suffering from hypertension or pre-hypertension.

These are only some of the reasons why the DASH Diet is very popular and why it has been ranked as the number 1 diet by the US News and World report for 5 years, namely 2011, 2012, 2013, 2014 and 2015. It is also recommended by multiple groups and associations such as "The National Heart, Lung and Blood Institute," "The American Heart Association," "The Dietary Guidelines for Americans," and "US Guidelines for Treating High Blood Pressure."

In 2017, the DASH Diet was also ranked yet again as the best diet for the 7th year in a row once again by the US News and World Report.

CHAPTER 2: HOW TO BE ON A SUCCESSFUL DASH DIET

Following a diet isn't that easy. Adopting a new one is even more difficult. It requires a tremendous amount of patience and discipline to pull off. It takes a lot of guts and adjustments to make a new healthy habit. Proper diets do not just last for 1 or 2 weeks more so less than that. At least a new eating regime gets noticeable positive change by 4 or 5 weeks. Starting and finishing a proper diet takes at the very least a month and can reach a few years or even more. In this chapter, you will learn tips on how it will be easier for you to follow the DASH Diet and eventually become a healthier and stronger you. Sounds good right? Here are some tips that you can do to kick-start your new DASH Diet easily.

Tip 1: Consult your doctor regularly. (Know what you can get from it)

It is not true that anyone can do all diets and that all foods are healthy. Sometimes taking on a specific diet may cause more harm than good to a person if he or she undergoes that process. So the best thing to do before you start dieting is to consult your doctor. There is nothing wrong with knowing more about your body. It is also most definitely better if you find out if the diet program will be beneficial or detrimental to your health. There are so many things to consider regarding what diet is best for a person such as your own goals, underlying condition, fat percentage, stress levels, and metabolism. Your doctor can find these things out for you and recommend you a more specific plan for your health like particular food and when to eat them. Even meditation can be recommended if you are a stressed individual and it has affected your diet. Although it may sound like a spoon-feeding step, it would make it easier for you to begin your new diet when you are equipped with all the information you need. General guidelines may not work for your specific body type, lifestyle, goals, etc., so that is why it is best to be enlightened by your physician with a personalized diet plan with Dash Diet as its foundation.

Tip 2: Make food that you like eating

Whoever said that dieting had to be a terrible experience? Most people associate taking on a new healthy diet as some excruciating experience – not being able to eat anything tasty, being hungry all the time, feeling weak, not being ready to eat with friends and family, and being a tedious person in a group who orders the dull side of the menu. Well, only those who do not know how to be creative with their diets say that. There are hundreds of thousands of things that you could do to make your diet better and exciting. Just because you are eating healthy does not mean that it has to taste bad or it has to have no taste at all. If you put flavor into your diet meals, it will make it easier for you to continue dieting without falling out of motivation.

In addition to that, the DASH Diet comes with multiple recipes already prepared for you. Also, as previously mentioned, you can still take the option of making your recipe while still following the DASH Diet. Your confidence in your meals affects how enjoyable it is. If you keep having negative thoughts that the new food you are eating is not delicious or that you would rather have something else, then you would not taste its goodness. And your hesitation will reflect on your face, and people would start to believe that your new diet is putting you on punishment. Cheer up, be positive, and be strong. The taste may be entirely different at first, but it would not kill you – your whining would stress and kill your aspiration. So give the new meals a chance and cherish its taste before complaining or judging entirely that it tastes awful. You need to work on your positivity and mental prowess for everything in your life to go one direction towards your goal, which in this case is a healthier you.

Tip 3: Don't overthink about it (Routine)

Sometimes what makes dieting hard is the constant thought that you are dieting. It makes you feel as though you are "suffering" because you cannot eat or drink some of the things that you want or that you usually consume. In this case, it might be soft drinks or white rice or anything that was prescribed as a "do not eat" item. One way to deal with this is to stop yourself from thinking that you are dieting. Condition yourself to believe that the diet is a part of your daily life. Make it a routine. Soon after that, you will realize that you have been following the diet for so long, but you haven't thought about it anymore. It is also a right way of getting rid of bad eating habits.

According to research, it takes about 30 days to adopt a new practice. It may be difficult at first. However, most likely by the second week of repetitively doing a new diet, it would be more relaxed and more comfortable. The new routine would integrate into your own daily life. As you consistently perform such task every day, your brain and body become wired into that activity. The new diet becomes a part of your lifestyle. If you treat DASH Diet as something healthy and be calm about it instead of continually pressing yourself for changes and sharply observing discomforts, then this new program would always feel foreign to your body. And what happens if you keep conditioning your mind that something is alien? It would reject it. Your diet will fail, and your body goals would not be achieved if you keep thinking negatively about your new diet.

Tip 4: Follow the recipes

Are you afraid you would not be able to stick to your new diet? Often, fear comes from the unknown. If you do not have enough knowledge about DASH Diet, then it is not uncommon to doubt whether you can see yourself through it or not. However, as mentioned earlier, the DASH Diet comes with recipes that you can quickly follow for your dieting needs. If you do not know or enjoy cooking your recipes, then this will be the best thing to do. This tip is similar to the second tip in a way because it tells you to choose what you eat so that you will not easily give up on the diet just because you do not like the taste or you are getting tired of eating the same thing again and again. Besides, the recipes that the DASH Diet gives are delicious and nutritious. Naturally, with the new job you are trying with a.k.a Dash Diet, your brain exerts more effort to keep up with the change. If you had to do your research and extensively plan your new meals to cook, then you would get very exhausted. If the supposedly new healthy habit makes you stressed, then it would most likely be unsuccessful or have very delayed results. To enable you to maintain high energy in resuming your daily life along the new diet, you can just get yourself coached by the supplied DASH Diet recipes. If you have these to consult every day or weekly, then you would not need to tire yourself up in coming up with new dishes in line with the diet. You merely have to follow them, eat them, and smoothly go your way towards your health goals.

Tip 5: Make the change gradually

Have you ever heard the phrase "slowly but surely?" It is better to make gradual changes that make a drastic one. Your chances of achieving your health or body goals successfully are higher if you do things in relevance to your own pace and capability. For example, if you are planning to get on the new diet such as the DASH Diet, do not abruptly change your whole eating program right then and there unless you have this history of being very flexible and adaptable to change. Before your planned overall diet change, slowly add the essentials to this diet to your current diet. You may eat a few servings of fruits and veggies every day or assimilate other parts of the DASH Diet to your daily meals until you eat more of the DASH diet food and smaller of your current diet. Make the transition smooth and not shocking to your body and taste buds. Just add more and more of the DASH Diet meals every day until you get used to it or you feel strong enough to shift to the new diet entirely. Add more of these nutritious foods gradually to make it a regular habit. Just like what people say, some things go as fast as they came. So if you change your diet too quickly, you may change back to your old diet just as swiftly also. The key to successful dieting is consistency. You may be more able to stick to the program if you gradually adapt it.

Tip 6: Reward yourself for success and don't be too hard when you slip-up

The human brain works in a reward and punishment system. Usually, an individual will go for things that made him feel positive responses such as happiness, fulfillment, or pleasure. A person tends to avoid those that make him think negativity such as sadness, discomfort, anger, and pain. You can train yourself to regard successful dieting as a rewarding experience. For example, if you have consistently stuck to your new DASH Diet for the whole week, then maybe you can treat yourself to the movies, the spa, or go shopping by the weekend. Or you could consider having a little bit of a cheat day. If you do this, you could lessen the possible stress accompanied by this change of food intake. It will condition your mind that is committed to your diet and not letting go of it despite the initial discomforts is a very significant thing. On the other hand, if ever you fall short on the consistency on your new diet, then do not be too hard on yourself. Look at the situation objectively – where could have you possibly went wrong? Examine your circumstance, know your triggers, and plan on how to overcome another setback. Learn from this mistake, and come on stronger on achieving your goals.

Tip 7: Move and exercise

DASH Diet does work. However, if you want to get results sooner or see changes in your health and body faster, then it is advisable also to get your body moving. Like all diets present in the market, moving and exercising will significantly help you in achieving your goal. Having physical activities help in boosting your metabolism and lowering your blood pressure. Especially if you are the type of person who could overthink things or you are sensitive to the discomforts brought along by the changes in your diet, then it is best for you also regularly to exercise. Doing so can help declutter your mind and make you more resilient to changes and discomforts. With the endorphins released during exercise, you become stronger mentally and physically to take on any challenge. If the new diet can make you a bit down because you cannot eat sweets or fats as much as you used to, then exercising can help raise up your happy hormones and keep you off from feeling down.

Also, if you have been going to the gym, lifting some weights, going for a power run, or if you take walks in such peaceful sceneries or among people who are also trying to stay healthy – then you would feel more motivated. If you keep to your routine of school or work, then go back to your home to face your new diet and then think about what you are missing because of it, you would just feel miserable. Whereas, if you add exercise to your daily life, then you would have lesser time to self-pity or overthink things. Try to take a walk every morning. Make sure that you set aside a schedule as to when you will have your daily exercise. It does not need to be rigorous or extremely hard. The important thing is that you have physical activity. Why not try to use the stairs instead of the elevator when going to the office?

Tip 8: Look for people to join you

Both in doing a new diet plan or by starting to follow an exercise program, getting yourself a buddy proved to be effective. Unless you are uncomfortable with having a companion, this tip will be very useful in helping you continue dieting and getting healthier. How is dieting with other people help you ask? Well having other people join you, in general, is helpful because it gives you people who can support you in your efforts. You will have constant reassurance that what you are doing is worth it and that if you are having a hard time, you will have someone to help you get through it.

If you have a buddy with you, then it would not be straightforward to quit because your motivation and commitment are doubled by the two or more of you.

If you have someone to do something together, then it would be easier to stick to it. For example, if you do the DASH Diet along with a friend then you can go shopping for your food or prepare your meals together. By being not alone in this, it would seem less of work and more of something fun and exciting. Usually, people would look forward to activities done together by a friend or groups of friends. And so by doing the new diet with someone would make you look forward to getting yourselves healthy. Moreover, by introducing the DASH Diet to other people, you also become a good influence and help them grow healthier people in the process. Other than assisting yourself you have also helped other people in the process.

Sample Recipes

DASH Diet is recognized by the US Department of Agriculture to be among the healthiest eating plans available to people nowadays. DASH Diet has its effectiveness acknowledged along with veganism, vegetarianism, and the Mediterranean diet. DASH Diet has been referred to by some people as the Americanized counterpart of the Mediterranean diet. Similarly, they emphasize the proper consumption of unprocessed food, whole grains, and lean meats. What sets DASH Diet apart from other preexisting diet plans is that instead of being restrictive, it is more of inclusive. Instead of a strongly inhibiting amount of calorie intake, DASH Diet promotes it. The researchers and creators of DASH Diet formulated the eating plan with foods that the people are already eating or are commonly available for them so that it would be easier for them to manage and adopt instead of eating new food or those that are hard to find in local sources.

This is where you start! You can conveniently begin your DASH Diet and be sure that you can commit to it by taking in some of these sample recipes. All the tips mentioned earlier would come in handy along these recipes. The DASH Diet presents many different recipes ranging from appetizers to beverages to main course dishes to bread dishes to desserts. Pick out the ones that are closest to the food you have in your current diet. Surely you will be able to find something that you will enjoy eating.

1. Whole-grain Pizza Margherita

Ingredients

For the dough:

- 1 tsp of active dry yeast

- 3/4 cup of warm water

- ¾ cup of whole wheat flour

- 2 tbsps of barley flour

- 2 teaspoons of gluten

- 1 tbsp of oats

- 1 tbsp of olive oil

For the topping

- 2 ½ cups of spinach, chopped

- 2 ½ cups of tomatoes, sliced

- 1 tbsp of oregano (minced)

- 1 tbsp of garlic (minced)

- 1 tsp of black pepper

- 2 ounces of mozzarella, fresh

Directions

1. To make the dough, dissolve yeast in warm water, let sit 5 minutes. Mix dry ingredients. Add oil and water-yeast mixture. Knead for 10-15 minutes for best texture. An electric mixer is helpful, but not necessary.

2. Let dough rise in the refrigerator for a minimum of 1 hour.

3. Preheat oven to 450 F. out dough ball on floured surface to 1/4-inch thickness. Place dough on baking sheet or pizza peel. Top with spinach, tomatoes, basil, oregano, garlic, black pepper, and mozzarella. Bake for 10-12 minutes, or until cheese melts and crust

becomes crispy. Serve hot and enjoy.

2.   Beef Stroganoff

Ingredients

- 1/2 cup chopped onion

- 1/2 pound boneless beef round steak, cut 3/4-inch thick, all fat removed

- 4 cups uncooked yolk-less egg noodles

- 1/2 can fat-free cream of mushroom soup (undiluted)

- 1/2 cup of water

- 1 tablespoon all-purpose (plain) flour

- 1/2 teaspoon paprika

- 1/2 cup fat-free sour cream

Directions

1.   In a nonstick frying pan, sauté the onions over medium heat until they're translucent, about 5 minutes. Add the beef and continue to cook for

another 5 minutes or until the beef is tender and browned throughout. Drain well and set aside.

2. Fill a large pot 3/4 full with water and bring to a boil. Add the noodles and cook until al dente (tender), 10 to 12 minutes, or according to the package directions. Drain the pasta thoroughly.

3. In a saucepan, whisk together the soup, water, and flour over medium heat. Stir until the sauce thickens, about 5 minutes.

4. Add the soup mixture and paprika to the beef in the frying pan. Over medium heat, stir the mixture until warmed through. Remove from heat and add the sour cream. Stir until combined.

5. To serve, divide the pasta among the plates. Top with the beef mixture and serve immediately.

3. Potato Skin

Ingredients

- 2 medium russet potatoes

- Butter-flavored cooking spray

- 1 tablespoon minced fresh rosemary

- 1/8 teaspoon freshly ground black pepper

Directions

1. Preheat the oven to 375 F.

2. Wash the potatoes and pierce with a fork. Place in the oven and bake until the skins are crisp about 1 hour.

3. Carefully — potatoes will be very hot — cut the potatoes in half and scoop out the pulp, leaving about 1/8 inch of the potato flesh attached to the skin. Save the pulp for another use.

4. Spray the inside of each potato skin with butter-flavored cooking spray. Press in the rosemary and pepper.

5. Return the skins to the oven for 5 to 10 minutes. Serve immediately.

4. Raspberry Chocolate Scones

Ingredients

- 1 cup whole-wheat pastry flour

- 1 cup all-purpose flour

- 1 tablespoon baking powder

- 1/4 teaspoon baking soda

- 1/3 cup trans-fat-free buttery spread

- 1/2 cup fresh or frozen raspberries

- 1/4 cup miniature chocolate chips

- 1 cup plus 2 tablespoons plain fat-free yogurt

- 2 tablespoons honey

- 1/2 teaspoon sugar

- 1/4 teaspoon cinnamon

Directions

1. Mix flours, baking powder and baking soda in a large mixing bowl.

2. Cut in buttery spread until crumbly.

3. Add berries and chocolate chips. Mix gently.

4. Mix yogurt and honey in a small bowl.

5. Add yogurt mixture to flour mixture, mixing until just blended.

6. Place ball of dough on the countertop. Knead one or two times.

7. Roll into a 1/2-inch-thick circle.

8. Cut into 12 wedges.

9. Place on lightly greased baking sheet.

10. Mix sugar and cinnamon in a small bowl.

11. Sprinkle over top of scones.

12. Bake at 400 F for 10 to 12 minutes.

4. Seasonal Fruit Palette

Ingredients

- 1/4 teaspoon ground cinnamon

- 1/4 teaspoon sugar

- 2 cups frozen strawberries, unsweetened (thawed)

- 1/2 cup powdered sugar

- 1 star fruit, sliced

- 1 peach, pitted and sliced

- 1 pear, pitted and sliced

- 1 plum, pitted and sliced

- 1 kiwi, peeled and sliced

- Fresh mint leaves, for garnish

Directions

1.   In a small bowl, stir together the cinnamon and sugar. Set aside.

2.   In a food processor or blender, combine the strawberries and powdered sugar. Pulse until smooth.

3.   Pour onto chilled dessert plates that have a rim.

4.   Arrange the sliced fruit on top.

5.   Sprinkle with the cinnamon-sugar mixture.

6.   Garnish with fresh mint and serve immediately.

5. Rainbow Ice Pops

Ingredients

•   1 1/2 cups diced strawberries, cantaloupe and watermelon

•   1/2 cup blueberries

•   2 cups 100 percent apple juice (or another favorite juice)

•   6 paper cups (6-8 ounces each)

•   6 craft sticks

Directions

1. Mix the fruit and divide evenly into the paper cups.

2.   Pour 1/3 cup of juice into each paper cup.

3.   Place the cups on a level surface in the freezer.

4.   Freeze until partially frozen, approximately 1 hour.

5. Insert a craft stick into center of each pop. Freeze until firm.

6. Buffalo Chicken Salad Wrap

Ingredients

- 3-4 ounces of chicken breasts

- 2 whole chipotle peppers

- 1/4 cup white wine vinegar

- 1/4 cup low-calorie mayonnaise

- 2 stalks celery, diced

- 2 carrots, cut into matchsticks

- 1 small yellow onion, diced (about 1/2 cup)

- 1/2 cup thinly sliced rutabaga or another root vegetable

- 4 ounces spinach, cut into strips

- 2 whole-grain tortillas (12-inch diameter)

Directions

1. You can use leftover or rotisserie chicken if you

have it. If not, preheat oven to 375 F or start the grill.

2.   Bake or grill chicken breasts for about 10 minutes on each side until interior temperature is 165 F.

3.   Remove, cool and cube chicken.

4.   In a blender, puree chipotle peppers with white wine vinegar and mayonnaise.

5.   Place all ingredients except spinach and tortillas in a bowl and mix thoroughly.

6.   Place 2 ounces spinach and half the mixture in each tortilla and wrap. Cut each wrap in half to serve.

7. White Chicken Chili

Ingredients

- 1 can (10 ounces) white chunk chicken

- 3 cups cooked white beans

- 1 can (14.5 ounces) low-sodium diced tomatoes

- 4 cups low-sodium chicken broth

- 1 medium onion, chopped

- 1/2 medium green pepper, chopped

- 1 medium red pepper, chopped

- 2 garlic cloves, minced

- 2 teaspoons chili powder

- 1 teaspoon ground cumin

- 1 teaspoon dried oregano

- Cayenne pepper, to taste

- 6 tablespoons shredded reduced-fat Monterey Jack cheese

- 3 tablespoons chopped fresh cilantro

- 6 ounces low-fat baked tortilla chips (about 65 chips)

Directions

1. In a large soup pot, add the chicken, beans, tomatoes and chicken broth. Cover and simmer over medium heat.

2. Meanwhile, spray a nonstick frying pan with cooking spray. Add the onions, peppers and garlic and sauté until the vegetables are soft, 3 to 5 minutes.

3. Add the onion and pepper mixture to the soup pot.

4. Stir in the chili powder, cumin, oregano and, as desired, cayenne pepper.

5. Simmer for about 10 minutes, or until all the vegetables are soft.

6.   Ladle into warmed bowls.

7.   Sprinkle each serving with 1 tablespoon cheese and 1 teaspoon cilantro.

8.   Serve with baked chips on the side (about 6 to 8 chips with each serving of chili).

8. Curried Cream of Tomato Soup with Apples

Ingredients

- 2 tablespoons olive oil

- 1 1/2 cups finely chopped onion

- 1 cup finely chopped celery

- 1 teaspoon minced garlic

- 1 tablespoon curry powder, or to taste

- 3 cups no-salt-added canned tomatoes, drained

- 1 bay leaf

- 1/2 teaspoon thyme

- Ground black pepper, to taste

- 1 cup long-grain brown rice

- 6 cups low-sodium vegetable or chicken broth

- 1 cup fat-free milk

- 1 1/2 cups apple cubes

Directions

1. In a soup pot, heat the oil over medium heat.

2. Add the chopped onion, celery and garlic.

3. Saute until tender, about 4 minutes.

4. Add the curry powder and cook, stirring about 1 minute.

5. Add the tomatoes, bay leaf, thyme, black pepper, and rice.

6. Stir constantly while bringing to a boil.

7. Add broth.

8. Return to boil and then simmer for about 30 minutes.

9. When rice is tender, remove the bay leaf.

10. Pour the soup into a food processor or

blender and puree until smooth.

11.   Pour the soup back into the pot and add the milk and apple cubes.

12.   Cook until heated through.

13. Ladle into individual warmed bowls and serve immediately.

9. Shrimp Ceviche

Ingredients

- 1/2 pound raw shrimp, cut in 1/4-inch pieces

- 2 lemons, zest, and juice

- 2 limes, zest, and juice

- 2 tablespoons olive oil

- 2 teaspoons cumin

- 1/2 cup diced red onion

- 1 cup diced tomato

- 2 tablespoons minced garlic

- 1 cup black beans, cooked

- 1/4 cup diced serrano chili pepper and seeds removed

- 1 cup diced cucumber, peeled and seeded

- 1/4 cup chopped cilantro

Directions

1.   Place shrimp in a shallow pan and cover with juice from the lemon and lime, reserving the zest.

2.   Refrigerate for at least 3 hours or until shrimp is firm and white.

3.   Mix remaining ingredients in separate bowl and set aside while shrimp is cold cooking.

4.   When ready to serve, mix shrimp and citrus juice with remaining ingredients.

5.   Serve with baked tortilla chips.

Recommended food servings

If you are the type who likes to create your dishes, then feel free to use your creativity. Aside from the healthy recipes, here are the essentials of DASH Diet that you can use as guidelines in preparing your meals. Listed below are some suggestions from the DASH Diet and what portions you can follow:

Grains: 6 to 8 servings a day

• Grains include bread, cereal, rice, and pasta. Examples of one serving of grains include 1 slice whole-wheat bread, 1 ounce (oz.) dry cereal, or 1/2 cup cooked cereal, rice or pasta.

• Focus on whole grains because they have more fiber and nutrients than do refined grains. For instance, use brown rice instead of white rice, whole-wheat pasta instead of regular pasta and whole-grain bread instead of white bread. Look for products labeled "100 percent whole grain" or "100 percent whole wheat."

• Grains are naturally low in fat, so avoid spreading on butter or adding cream and cheese sauces.

Vegetables: 4 to 5 servings a day

• Tomatoes, carrots, broccoli, sweet potatoes, greens and other vegetables are full of fiber, vitamins, and such minerals as potassium and magnesium. Examples of one serving include 1 cup raw leafy green vegetables or 1/2 cup cut-up raw or cooked vegetables.

• Don't think of vegetables only as side dishes — a hearty blend of vegetables served over brown rice or whole-wheat noodles can serve as the main dish for a meal.

• Fresh or frozen vegetables are both good choices. When buying frozen and canned vegetables, choose those labeled as low sodium or without added salt.

• To increase the number of servings, you fit in daily, be creative. In a stir-fry, for instance, cut the amount of meat in half and double up on the vegetables.

Fruits: 4 to 5 servings a day

•   Many fruits need little preparation to become a healthy part of a meal or snack. Like vegetables, they're packed with fiber, potassium, and magnesium and are typically low in fat — exceptions include avocados and coconuts. Examples of one serving include 1 medium fruit or 1/2 cup fresh, frozen or canned fruit or 4 ounces of juice.

•   Have a piece of fruit with meals and one as a snack, then round out your day with a dessert of fresh fruits topped with a splash of low-fat yogurt.

•   Leave on edible peels whenever possible. The peels of apples, pears and most fruits with pits add interesting texture to recipes and contain healthy nutrients and fiber.

• Remember that citrus fruits and juice, such as grapefruit, can interact with certain medications, so check with your doctor or pharmacist to see if they're OK with you.

• If you choose can fruit or juice, make sure no sugar is added.

Dairy: 2 to 3 servings a day

• Milk, yogurt, cheese and other dairy products are major sources of calcium, vitamin D, and protein. But the key is to make sure that you choose dairy products that are low fat or fat-free because otherwise, they can be a major source of fat — and most of it is saturated. Examples of one serving include 1 cup skim or 1 percent milk, 1 cup yogurt, or 1 1/2 oz. Cheese.

• Low-fat or fat-free frozen yogurt can help you boost the number of dairy products you eat while offering a sweet treat. Add fruit for a healthy twist.

• If you have trouble digesting dairy products, choose lactose-free products or consider taking an over-the-counter product that contains the enzyme lactase, which can reduce or prevent the symptoms of lactose intolerance.

• Go easy on regular and even fat-free cheeses because they are typically high in sodium.

Lean meat, poultry, and fish: 6 or fewer servings a day

• Meat can be a rich source of protein, B vitamins, iron, and zinc. But because even lean varieties contain fat and cholesterol, don't make them a mainstay of your diet — cut back typical meat portions by one-third or one-half and pile on the vegetables instead. Examples of one serving include 1 oz. Cooked skinless poultry, seafood or lean meat or 1 egg.

• Trim away skin and fat from poultry and meat and then bake, broil, grill or roast instead of frying in fat.

• Eat heart-healthy fish, such as salmon, herring, and tuna. These types of fish are high in omega-3 fatty acids, which can help lower your total cholesterol.

These suggestions are some of the servings directly quoted from the DASH Diet. What was presented here are well-balanced amounts of servings that will help you achieve your goal of either lowering blood pressure or cutting down some weight.

Change to a Healthier Lifestyle

Dieting alone would not fully make you a healthier person. Although having a good diet creates significant improvement in your health, there is still something you can do to be even better. Or if your new diet has not been making any progress then a few lifestyle changes are advisable. For example, if you have hypertension, the cause of your condition is not only from an unhealthy diet, but it is also affected by your habits. It just makes sense that you should change not only your eating program but your other practices as well to reduce or eliminate your hypertension. Here are a few gradual changes you could apply to your life:

• Water – drink a bit more of water every day. It is recommended to consume at least 2 liters of water daily. Limit or eradicate at all drinking sugar-sweetened beverages such as sodas, chocolate drinks, sugary shakes, coffee, and the like.

• Drinking – lessen your alcohol intakes especially that most drinking sessions are associated with other unhealthy habits

• Smoking – lessen your smoking habit until you can entirely quit it. Stay away from individuals smoking or from smoking areas as to not risk yourself from breathing secondhand smoke

• Sleep – get more sleep if you are not having enough, and get proper amount of sleep if you are having too much

• Dessert – you can eat have fruits as dessert instead of the usual sugar-filled ones such as ice cream, chocolates, candies, cake, and other pastries. If you want to eat some sweets, eat in smaller portions.

• Salt – instead of using salt in your cooking, use herbs and spices instead. To avoid using salt or to limit its accessibility, do not put salt shakers on your dining table.

• Snacks – most individuals opt for salty and sweet snacks. When you start inching for another bag of potato chips or a box of doughnuts, have some fresh fruits instead. Another thing you can snack on are strips of vegetables. You can keep cut carrots, mixed greens, and bell peppers for a quick snack.

• Be more active – at least spare 10 minutes a day to exercise like walking, taking the stairs, bicycling, jogging, etc. If you can, it is better to have at least 30 minutes of work out for four to five times a week.

• Exercise plan – plot yourself an exercise plan or get yourself a work out buddy or a personal trainer to be able to stick to keeping yourself fit.

• Health check – regularly consult your physician instead of only taking a trip to the clinic if you are sick or unwell. It is best to have your blood pressure, blood cholesterol, and glucose levels checked timely.

It is not easy to make an abrupt change in your lifestyle. So try to apply one or two of them week by week until you form a habit of it. In no time, you would get used to having such healthy lifestyle, and you would just naturally be such a healthy individual.

CHAPTER 3: THE REWARDS THAT YOU WILL REAP

With the DASH Diet having its foundation on health rather than vanity, there are so many benefits that you can get when following the diet. Below are some of its great rewards to help you further understand and take that first step to changing your life for the better.

Prevention of Diabetes

It is estimated that in the United States of America alone there are 29.1 million people who have diabetes. Out of that 29.1 million 8.1 million of them may be undiagnosed or unaware of their current condition. In adults 20 and older, more than one in every 10 people suffers from diabetes, and in seniors (65 and older), that figure rises to more than one in four. Diabetes is not something to be taken lightly. A person who is affected by this condition can experience getting damage to the large blood vessels of the brain, heart or legs. Damage to the small blood vessels is also possible; this can cause problems to the eyes, kidneys, feet, and nerves. Right now there is still no cure for diabetes. With this in mind, the best thing to do is to follow the saying; "prevention is better than a cure."

There are two main types of diabetes; Type 1 and Type 2. The difference between the two is basically how they are acquired, but they have the same effect. Diabetes is caused by the increase of glucose in the blood which in turn is caused by the lack of insulin or possibly the body not responding properly to the insulin which is already present. This is where the DASH Diet plays its role. According to a study conducted by Angela D. Liese, PhD, MPH, Michele Nichols, MS, Xuezheng Sun, MSPH, Ralph B. D'Agostino, Jr., PhD and Steven M. Haffner, MD wherein they associated the occurrence of type 2 diabetes in people from different races and places and with different genders whom all followed the

Dash Diet. They were able to conclude from their study that the Dash Diet may indeed prove beneficial to the prevention of diabetes.

Since this diet promotes the improvement of insulin sensitivity it also helps prevent the occurrence of diabetes in the person who follows it. According to multiple studies that tackled the effects of diet accompanied by different degrees of exercise on the occurrence of diabetes, "Previous randomized trials of lifestyle interventions have demonstrated that increasing physical activity combined with a diet to encourage weight loss can decrease the incidence of type 2 diabetes in susceptible individuals...Diet interventions focused on caloric restriction, reduced fat intake, and increased fiber consumption. Overall, the exercise plus diet interventions resulted in significant weight loss and reduced the risk of diabetes by 37%." About the DASH Diet specifically, it is clear that it is under this category since the diet will also tell you to lower your fat and sodium intake and only eat good carbohydrates rich in fiber and many other things.

On Weight Loss

Losing weight is possible when there is lesser calorie count in one's body. The DASH Diet, however, do not emphasize on reducing calorie intake. It suggests nutrient-dense foods instead of calorie-rich ones to lose some inches off the waist. Fiber-rich diet proved to be effective in losing weight.

The best way to be healthy is to have a well-balanced diet which is at the same time packed with nutrients. And the DASH Diet is absolutely that. Due to its malleability, it allows for a successful and sustainable dieting. It does not leave the body deprived and hungry, unlike other diet plans. It merely reduces the number of processed fats and sweets and reimburses with fruits, vegetables, and low-fat dairy produce. Although the DASH Diet was initially created to lower blood pressure, it is also beneficial for losing weight. It is due to its eating plan that involves real foods with the right proportion of proteins, and with lots of fruits and vegetables. Because it is healthy and smooth at the same time, it is applicable throughout one's life. It is also not restrictive on adults or individuals who have health conditions, but anyone can eat it including the kids or the whole family. With DASH diet as the household's healthy meal plan, there would be lesser or no need at all for anyone to watch their diet. This is very beneficial for individuals who are gaining weight due to metabolic syndrome, type 2 diabetes, PCOS, and postmenopausal weight gain.

Hypertension

Dash in DASH Diet means Dietary Approaches to Stop Hypertension. In the U.S. alone, hypertension affects over fifty million people. Internationally, individuals who have high blood pressure reach up to 1 billion. Reportedly by the World Health

Organization, hypertension causes approximately 7.1 million deaths yearly. Hypertension is a severe case since it does not only affect one's blood pressure but it affects or causes other conditions in one's body. It induces a heart attack, stroke, heart failure, and even kidney disease. By eating the DASH Diet and sparing yourself from hypertension, you are also keeping yourself away from other circulatory and excretory diseases.

To give you a glimpse of what is a healthy blood pressure and when you should start to worry, here is a bit of an explanation regarding normal blood pressure. There are two numbers recorded as blood pressure is taken – one is systolic, and another one is diastolic. The name on top is systolic, while the bottom one is diastolic. Systolic is usually higher than diastolic. It measures the pressure in the arteries as the muscles in the heart contracts or heartbeat. On the other hand, diastolic is the number that measures the pressure in the arteries in between muscle contraction in the heart or when it is resting or refilling blood. The normal range for systolic pressure is 120 or below while the normal range for diastolic pressure is 80 or lower. So numbers higher than these imply tendency of having hypertension.

Osteoporosis

Another health benefit to DASH Diet is sparing you from having osteoporosis. It is a disease where the body produces too much or too little bones or losses bones. It is quite common among elderly individuals. The new DASH Diet can help you avoid suffering from this illness. The diet is rich in calcium, protein, and potassium which are all necessary for preventing or slowing down osteoporosis. Food such as milk, lean meat, grains, leafy vegetables, and fruits help build stronger bones. See yourself as a healthy older adult with good posture if you start eating the DASH Diet as soon as possible.

Kidney Health

Kidney problems are among the most common diseases that individuals nowadays have – from urinary tract infections (UTI), kidney stones, to kidney failure. These are caused by excessive mineral deposits in the kidneys that form into stones. It makes urinating very painful. It also creates other bodily pains such as intense backaches. High mineral deposits in one's kidneys result from high sodium intake which dehydrates the body and overworks the kidneys. DASH Diet includes lowering of sodium in one's meals, which ultimately makes it very helpful in the prevention of and recovery from kidney problems.

Cancer Prevention

One the diseases that people fear the most is cancer. Cancer is somewhat unpredictable since it could happen to anyone. However, the chances of getting one can be lowered by adopting the DASH Diet. The high concentration of fiber, vitamins, and antioxidants in fruits, vegetables, and whole grains in the DASH Diet lessens or stops altogether the effect of free radicals. One of them is the byproducts of cellular respiration. This causes mutation in healthy cells which can lead to cancer.

CONCLUSION

Undoubtedly, the DASH Diet is by far the most effective and useful eating program not just for those with body conditions but for those who are aiming to cut some pounds off their body. There are so many benefits one can get when eating the DASH Diet. Despite it being a new eating program, it proves to be less difficult to adapt to, unlike other preexisting diets. DASH Diet is very beneficial to individuals of all ages, even to the whole family. Among its main purposes are to help with:

• Hypertension or high blood pressure

• Diabetes

• Weight loss

Additionally, it is great for the alleviation and prevention of osteoporosis, kidney problems, and cancer. DASH Diet is a very nutritious eating program. To sum up, its general idea on how to eat a healthy diet, take this in mind:

• Grains and grain products: 6 to 8 servings include at least three whole grain foods such as sliced bread, dry cereal, cooked cereal, pasta, rice, or barley

- Fruits: 4 to 5 servings such as grapefruits, banana, raisins, dried fruits

- Vegetables: 4 to 5 servings such as spinach leaves, peppers, sliced tomatoes, sprouts, zucchini, portobello mushrooms, and eggplant

- Low- or non-fat dairy foods: 2 to 3 servings such as 1% to nonfat milk, low-fat yogurt, and cheese

- Lean meats, fish, poultry: 6 or less such as fresh chicken breast or legs, fresh turkey breast, loin cuts of beef, sirloin, round steak, extra-lean ground beef, pork loin roast, pork tenderloin, fresh fish, and low-sodium canned tuna

- Nuts, seeds, and legumes: 4 to 5 servings per week such as nut butter, unsalted sunflower seeds

- Healthy Fats: 2 to 3 servings such as olive, peanut, canola oils, soybean oil, and corn oil

- Sweets: 2 or fewer such as a 2-inch square brownie, a

small donut, a miniature candy bar, 2 small cookies, 1 small muffin, and 1 small piece of pie or cake

By sticking to this diet, you will naturally be consuming lesser salt. If you cannot follow the suggested recipe samples in this book and you want to cook the same dishes you are used to preparing; you can limit your sodium intake by simply putting less or no salt at all on the meals you cook. Also, it would help to remove the salt shakers on your dining table, so you do not keep on adding salt to your meals. Another thing to watch besides your sodium intake is your alcohol consumption. Males should cut down their liquor to at most 2 drinks per day while females should limit herself to only one. By controlling one's alcohol consumption, one's weight would be managed better, blood pressure will be normal, and dehydration would be less likely to occur.

This DASH Diet book gives you everything you need to know to successfully be a healthier you. Besides giving you actual recipes you can use while you are still new with the diet, the book also suggested lifestyle changes you can make to be healthier, and also to aid the progress that the DASH Diet will bring upon your body. Remember these healthy habits that you should gradually incorporate into your daily life.

•	Drink more water every day and cut back on sweetened and alcoholic drinks

•	Quit smoking or stay away from secondhand smoke

•	Snack on fruits and vegetables and just eat little portions of sweets and fats

•	Use herbs and spices instead of salt; do not put salt shakers on your dining table to avoid adding more salt to your meals

•	Exercise at least 10 minutes a day if you are really busy like taking the stairs, walking, or riding the bicycle

•	Get a workout buddy or personal trainer so that you can do at least 30 minutes of exercise 4 to 5 times a week

•	Consult with your doctor regularly

Your goal of achieving a healthier you is within your reach. DASH Diet is your best choice in going towards this aspiration. Unlike other diets, DASH Diet is directed towards preventing or alleviating certain body conditions instead of focusing on just losing weight to look good. Aim towards your core health first, and then your vigor will manifest outside with a fit body. You are not left alone to struggle hard with your initial attempt on DASH Diet because even from this book alone, you are furnished recipes and guidelines that you can use for your daily new healthy lifestyle. Try it out for a week or so, and you will know how easy it is. For sure you would quickly progress to a second, third, up to a fourth week, and up to a whole healthy lifetime.

FINAL WORDS

Thank you again for purchasing this book! I really hope this book is able to help you.

The next step is for you to **join our email newsletter** to receive updates on any upcoming new book releases or promotions. You can sign-up for free and as a bonus, you will also receive our "*7 Fitness Mistakes You Don't Know You're Making*" book! This bonus book breaks down many of the most common fitness mistakes and will demystify many of the complexities and science of getting into shape. Having all this fitness knowledge and science organized into an actionable step-by-step book will help you get started in the right direction in your fitness journey! To join our free email newsletter and grab your free book, please visit the link and signup: **www.hmwpublishing.com/gift**

Finally, if you enjoyed this book, then I would like to ask you for a favor, would you be kind enough to leave a review for this book? It would be greatly appreciated!

Thank you and good luck in your journey!

ABOUT THE CO-AUTHOR

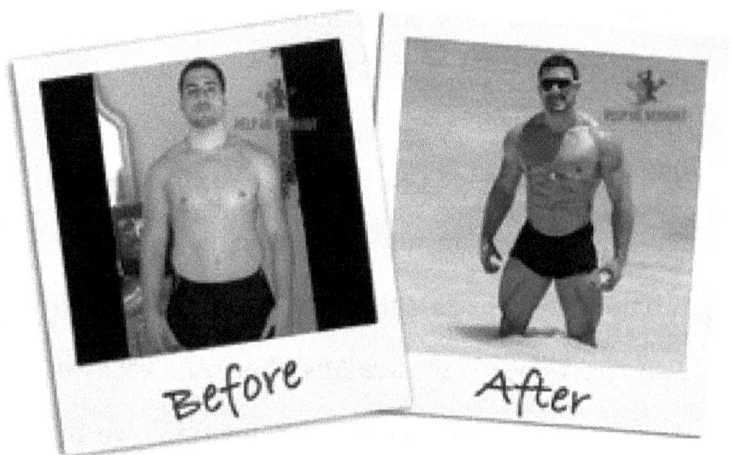

Before After

My name is George Kaplo; I'm a certified personal trainer from Montreal, Canada. I'll start off by saying I'm not the biggest guy you will ever meet and this has never really been my goal. In fact, I started working out to overcome my biggest insecurity when I was younger, which was my self-confidence. This was due to my height measuring only 5 foot 5 inches (168cm), it pushed me down to attempt anything I ever wanted to achieve in life. You may be going through some challenges right now, or you may simply want to get fit, and I can certainly relate.

For me personally, I was always kind of interested in the health & fitness world and wanted to gain some muscle due to the numerous bullying in my teenage years about my height and my overweight body. I figured I couldn't do anything about my height, but I sure can do something about how my body looked like. This was the beginning of my transformation journey. I had no idea where to start, but I just got started. I felt worried and afraid at times that other people would make fun of me for doing the exercises the wrong way. I always wished I had a friend that was next to me who was knowledgeable enough to help me get started and "show me the ropes."

After a lot of work, studying and countless trial and errors. Some people began to notice how I was getting more fit and how I was starting to form a keen interest in the topic. This led many friends and new faces to come to me and ask me for fitness advice. At first, it seemed odd when people asked me to help them get in shape. But what kept me going is when they started to see changes in their own body and told me it's the first time that they saw real results!

From there, more people kept coming to me, and it made me realize after so much reading and studying in this field that it did help me but it also allowed me to help others. I'm now a fully certified personal trainer and have trained numerous clients to date who have achieved amazing results.

Today, my brother Alex Kaplo (also a Certified Personal Trainer) and I own & operate this publishing venture, where we bring passionate and expert authors to write about health and fitness topics. We also run an online fitness website "HelpMeWorkout.com" and I would love to connect with by inviting you to visit the website on the following page and signing up to our e-mail newsletter (you will even get a free book). Last but not least, if you are in the position I was once in and you want some guidance, don't hesitate and ask... I'll be there to help you out!

Your friend and coach,

George Kaplo
Certified Personal Trainer

Get another book for Free

I want to thank you for purchasing this book and offer you another book (just as long and valuable as this book), "Health & Fitness Mistakes You Don't Know You're Making", completely free.

Visit the link below to signup and receive it:

www.hmwpublishing.com/gift

In this book, I will break down the most common health & fitness mistakes, you are probably committing right now, and I will reveal how you can easily get in the best shape of your life!

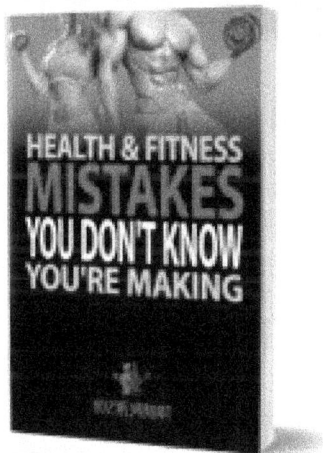

In addition to this valuable gift, you will also have an opportunity to get our new books for free, enter giveaways, and receive other valuable emails from me. Again, visit the link to sign up:

www.hmwpublishing.com/gift

Copyright 2017 by HMW Publishing - All Rights Reserved.

This document by HMW Publishing owned by the A&G Direct Inc company, is geared towards providing exact and reliable information in regards to the topic and issue covered. The publication is sold with the idea that the publisher is not required to render accounting, officially permitted, or otherwise, qualified services. If advice is necessary, legal or professional, a practiced individual in the profession should be ordered.

From a Declaration of Principles which was accepted and approved equally by a Committee of the American Bar Association and a Committee of Publishers and Associations.

In no way is it legal to reproduce, duplicate, or transmit any part of this document in either electronic means or in printed format. Recording of this publication is strictly prohibited, and any storage of this document is not allowed unless with written permission from the publisher. All rights reserved.

The information provided herein is stated to be truthful and consistent, in that any liability, in terms of inattention or otherwise, by any usage or abuse of any policies, processes, or directions contained within is the solitary and utter responsibility of the recipient reader. Under no circumstances will any legal responsibility or blame be held against the publisher for any reparation, damages, or monetary loss due to the information herein, either directly or indirectly.

The information herein is offered for informational purposes solely, and is universal as so. The presentation of the information is without contract or any type of guarantee assurance.

The trademarks that are used are without any consent, and the publication of the trademark is without permission or backing by the trademark owner. All trademarks and brands within this book are for clarifying purposes only and are the owned by the owners themselves, not affiliated with this document.

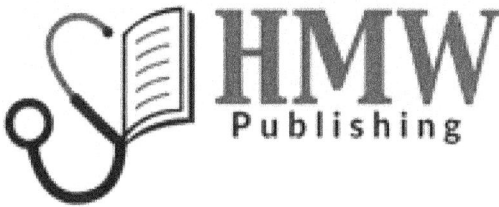

For more great books visit:

HMWPublishing.com

www.ingramcontent.com/pod-product-compliance
Lightning Source LLC
Chambersburg PA
CBHW071246020426
42333CB00015B/1650

9781999283353